# The Phoenix Journey Cookbook: Vol 1

Eating For Your Autoimmune Journey | Beyond The Pill

*To the incredible Phoenix Journey community and all the autoimmune warriors who continue to fight with strength and resilience—this book is for you. May you always remember that even in the darkest moments, there is hope and healing waiting to be found. Rise up from the ashes, embrace your power and your journey. Together, we are unstoppable.*

# About the Author

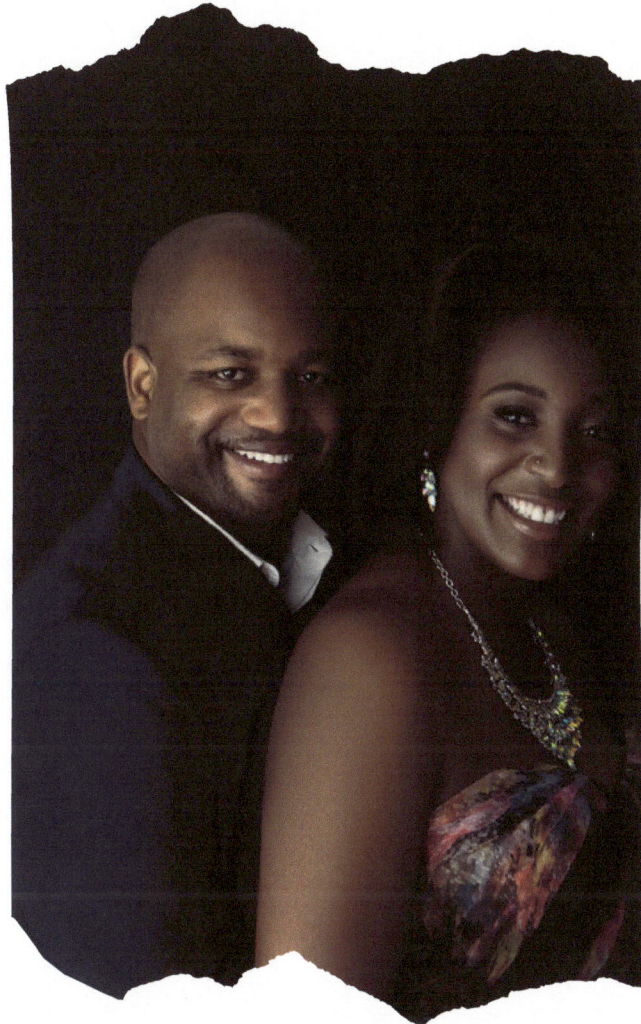

Dominique is a resilient survivor, diagnosed with severe form of active Primary Progressive Multiple Sclerosis, which left her in a wheelchair with little hope. However, with the unwavering support, her husband, the renowned Chef Adrian, she embarked on a journey to reclaim her health. Chef Adrian inspired by their shared experience, crafted healing dishes that transformed her health and helped the autoimmune community. Inspired by her journey, Dominique founded The Phoenix Journey to empower others facing similar challenges. Together, they continue to reshape the way food is seen as medicine, changing lives across the country, just as Dominique has.

# **Welcome to Your Path to Healing: A Cookbook for Autoimmune Health**

Living with an autoimmune disease can feel like navigating a world where the body's natural defenses seem to be working against you. Whether you're newly diagnosed or have been living with an autoimmune condition for years, managing the symptoms and improving your quality of life requires a holistic approach—one that includes not only medical care but also a careful, nurturing diet.

This cookbook is designed specifically for those who are navigating the challenges of autoimmune disease. It provides a collection of nourishing recipes that are both healing and delicious, crafted to support your body's natural healing processes while helping you manage inflammation, gut health, and immune function. Every meal you prepare here is more than just food—it is a step toward feeling better, supporting your immune system, and taking control of your health.

### Understanding Autoimmune Health

Autoimmune diseases occur when the immune system mistakenly attacks the body's own cells, leading to inflammation, pain, and other symptoms that can impact every area of life. Some of the most common autoimmune conditions include eczema, rheumatoid arthritis, lupus, multiple sclerosis, type 1 diabetes, Hashimoto's thyroiditis, celiac disease, and Crohn's disease, among others. These diseases can cause a variety of symptoms, from fatigue and joint pain to digestive issues and brain fog. While there is no one-size-fits-all treatment, managing your diet is an important tool for controlling symptoms and improving overall health.

# Key Facts About Autoimmune Health:

1. **Inflammation**: Many autoimmune conditions are characterized by chronic inflammation. This inflammation can be influenced by the foods we eat, so making anti-inflammatory choices is key to managing flare-ups.

2. **Gut Health**: There is growing evidence that gut health plays a significant role in autoimmune diseases. A balanced, diverse gut microbiome can support the immune system, while an imbalance may trigger or worsen symptoms.

3. **Food Sensitivities**: Certain foods, such as gluten, dairy, and processed sugars, are known to aggravate autoimmune symptoms in many individuals. This cookbook helps you navigate food sensitivities by focusing on nutrient-dense, healing foods that support your body's natural function.

4. **The Power of Nourishing Ingredients**: Healing ingredients—such as turmeric, ginger, leafy greens, and healthy fats—have powerful anti-inflammatory properties and provide essential nutrients that are often deficient in those with autoimmune conditions. By incorporating these into your meals, you're fueling your body to heal itself.

### Why This Cookbook is Different

This cookbook isn't just about making food—it's about healing through food. Every recipe is designed with autoimmune health in mind, focusing on nourishing your body, supporting your immune system, and reducing inflammation. Whether you are looking for simple meals to ease digestive discomfort or recipes to support joint health, this cookbook offers a variety of options to fit your unique needs.

What sets this cookbook series apart is the attention to the specific dietary requirements that are vital for autoimmune health. You will see between this book and the rest of the volumes:
- **Anti-inflammatory ingredients** to help combat pain and inflammation.
- **Gluten-free, dairy-free, and low-sugar** options that are carefully curated for those with sensitivities.
- **Gut-healing recipes** that feature ingredients like bone broth, fermented foods, and prebiotic-rich vegetables.
- **Adaptable meals** that can cater to different autoimmune conditions and personal preferences, offering versatility and ease for your healing journey.

By using this cookbook, you are taking proactive steps toward reclaiming control over your health. The recipes provided will not only help manage the symptoms of autoimmune disease but will also help you reconnect with food as a source of nourishment and empowerment.

Whether you are making a quick breakfast or preparing a healing dinner, this cookbook will guide you with ease, offering practical solutions that fit into your daily life. You deserve to feel your best, and with the right nourishment, it's possible.

Let this cookbook be your companion on a journey of healing, self-care, and renewal.

# Blueberry Muffins

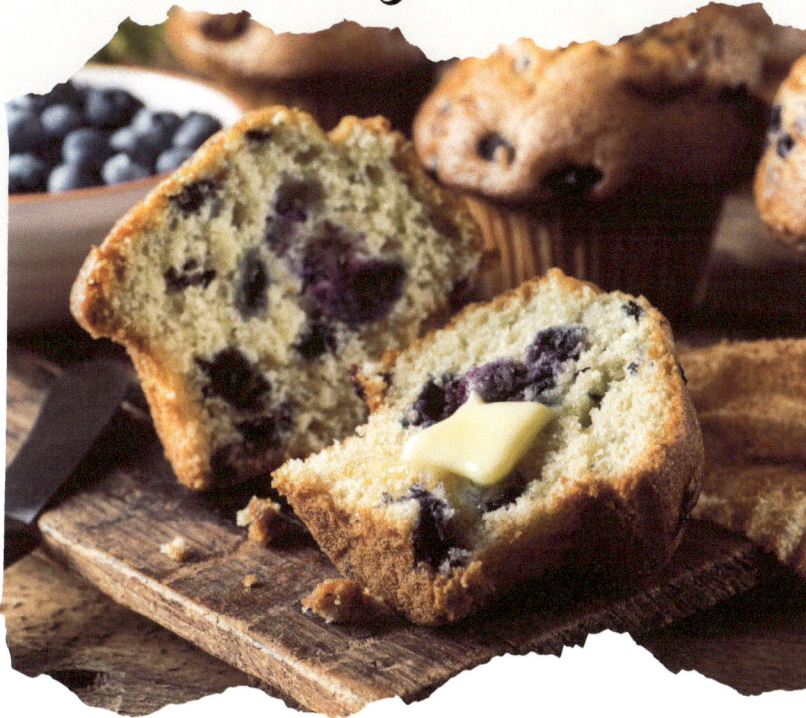

*This image may not be an accurate representation of the recipe.*

## Ingredients

- 3 small or 2 large bananas
- 1/4 cup apple butter
- 2 eggs lightly beaten
- 2 cups Almond flour
- 1 tsp Baking powder
- 1 pint Blueberries
- 2 tsp Vanilla
- 1/2 tsp Salt

## Method

1. Preheat Oven: Preheat oven to 350 degrees and line muffin pan with muffin liners.
2. Mix Wet Ingredients: Smash bananas in a bowl with a fork and add apple butter, egg and vanilla and mix well.
3. Mix In Dry Ingredients: Sprinkle baking soda in the wet mix and whisk; add almond flour and whisk together.
4. Fold In Blueberries: Add the blueberries and fold in gently
5. Bake: Bake 18-20 min until a toothpick comes out clean
6. Rest: Rest muffins on a cooling rack for 5 minutes

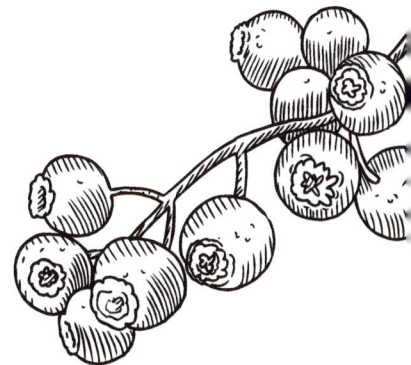

# Migas

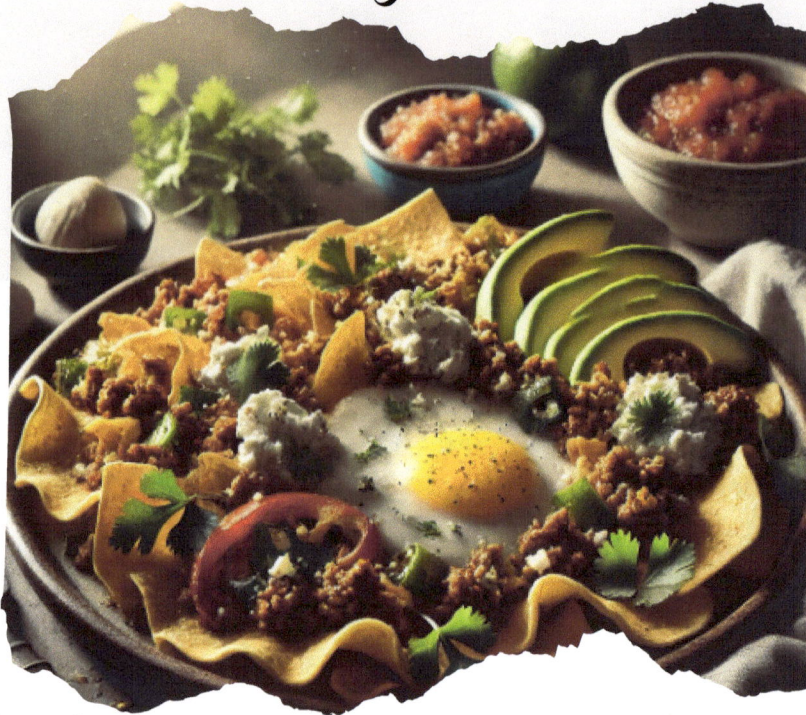

*This image may not be an accurate representation of the recipe.

## Ingredients

2 Tablespoons Avocado or olive oil

1 Small Onion

1 Small Bell pepper

3 Cloves of Garlic

1/2 pound ground beef

Siete tortillas cut in 6

1 Tablespoon Cumin

1 Tablespoon Chili powder

2 Teaspoons Chicken Knorr seasoning

Salt and pepper to taste

6 Eggs

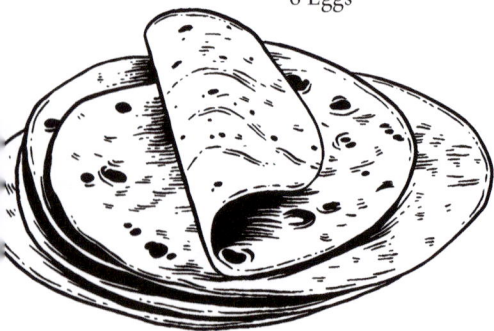

## Method

1. Prepare Tortillas: Cut the tortillas into six or triangles

2. Fry the Tortillas: Heat 2 tablespoons of avocado or olive oil in a large skillet over medium heat. Add the tortilla pieces and fry them until crispy and golden brown, about 2-4 minutes.  Flip halfway through to avoid burning. Once crispy, remove them from the skillet and set them aside on a paper towel to drain excess oil.

3. Cook the Beef: In the same skillet, add the ground beef. Cook over medium heat, breaking it apart with a spatula until browned and cooked through. Drain any excess fat.

4. Add Veggies and Spices: Add the chopped onion, bell pepper, and garlic to the skillet with the beef. Cook for 3-4 minutes, until softened. Stir in the cumin, chili powder, salt, and pepper, cooking for another minute to toast the spices.

5. Scramble the Eggs: Push the beef and veggies to one side of the skillet and crack the eggs into the empty side. Scramble the eggs, and when slightly wet, add the crispy tortilla pieces back into the skillet and mix until everything is well combined.

6. Serve: Once everything is mixed, taste and adjust the seasoning with more salt and pepper if needed. Serve with your choice of optional toppings, like salsa, avocado, goat cheese, or cilantro.

# Fried Brown Rice with Cauliflower Rice

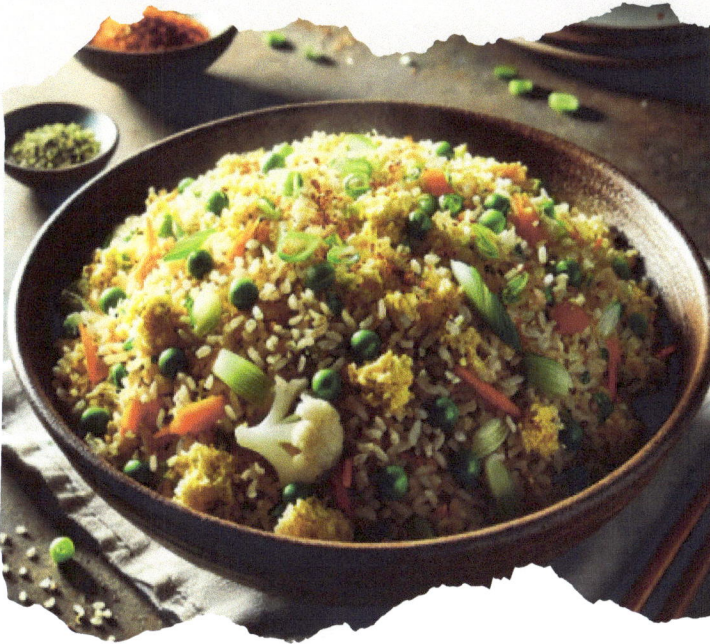

*This image may not be an accurate representation of the recipe.

## Ingredients

1 cup Cooked and cooled brown rice

1/2 cup minced carrots

1/2 cup minced celery

2 cups cauliflower rice

1/4 cup Sesame oil

1 1/2 cup Coconut aminos

2 tbsp Garlic powder

1 tsp ground ginger

1 cup peas

4 Eggs beaten

## Method

**1.Prepare the Rice:** If you haven't already, cook the brown rice and let it cool completely (or use leftover rice).

**2.Cook the Vegetables:** Heat 1 tablespoon of oil in a large skillet or wok over medium-high heat.

Add the diced onion and sauté for about 2-3 minutes until soft.

Add the garlic, add red pepper flakes, and sauté for another 30 seconds until fragrant.

Add the peas and carrots (if frozen, no need to thaw) and cook for about 3-4 minutes until heated through.

**3.Scramble the Eggs:** Push the vegetables to one side of the pan and add a little more oil if needed. Pour the beaten eggs into the empty space and scramble them until fully cooked. Then, mix the eggs with the vegetables.

**4. Cook the Cauliflower Rice:** Add the cauliflower rice to the pan and stir-fry for 4-5 minutes until it softens slightly but still has some texture. Season with a pinch of salt, pepper, and ginger if using.

**5.Add the Brown Rice:** Add the cooked and cooled brown rice to the pan with the cauliflower rice and vegetables. Stir everything together to combine and heat through.

**6.Flavor:** Pour in the coconut aminos, stirring to evenly coat everything. Taste and adjust the seasoning, adding more coconut aminos or salt if needed.

**7.Serve:** Garnish with chopped green onions

Goes well with the Korean beef

For extra protein, add cooked chicken, beef or shrimp

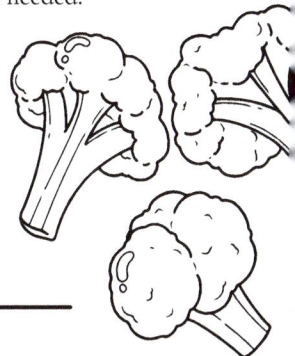

# Jalapeño Mango Grilled Chicken Breast

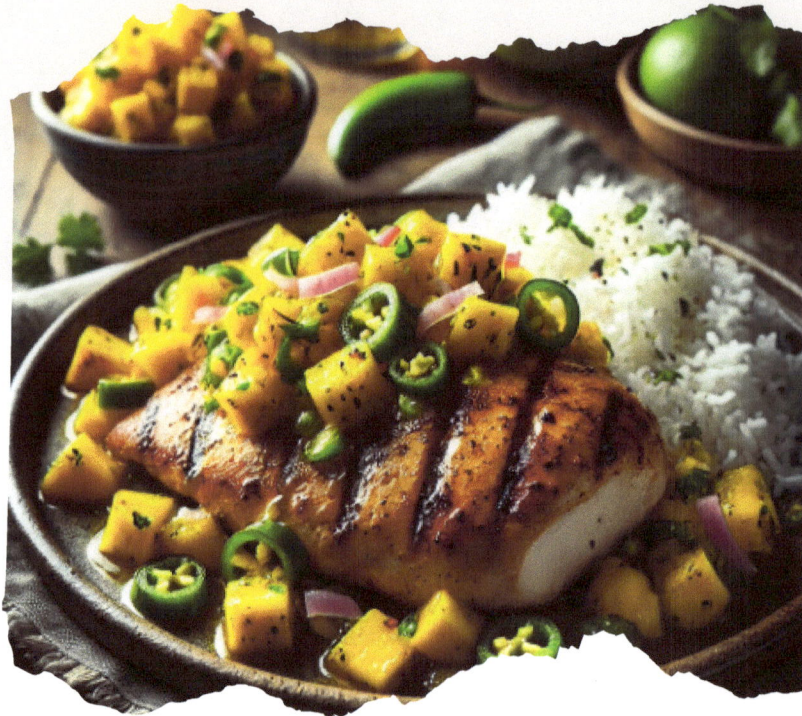

*This image may not be an accurate representation of the recipe.

## Ingredients

2 large boneless, skinless chicken breasts cut in half lengthwise or 4 small chicken breast

2 ripe mangos, peeled and diced

1-2 jalapeños, deseeded and finely chopped (adjust to taste)

1 small red onion, finely chopped

2 cloves garlic, minced

Apple cider vinegar ¼ cup

1 tablespoon fresh lime juice

1 tablespoon honey

1 tablespoon olive oil

Salt and pepper to taste

Fresh cilantro for garnish (optional)

## Method

1.**Prepare the Chicken:** Season the chicken breasts with salt and pepper on both sides. Heat olive oil in a large skillet over medium heat. Cook the chicken breasts for 5-6 minutes on each side or until fully cooked through 165°F. Remove the chicken from the skillet and set aside.

2.**Make the Jalapeno Mango Salsa:** In the same skillet, add the chopped red onion and cook for about 2 minutes until softened. Use more oil if needed. Add the garlic and chopped jalapeños to the pan and cook for another 1-2 minutes until fragrant. Stir in the diced mango, lime juice, apple cider vinegar, and honey. Cook for another 3-4 minutes, stirring occasionally, until the mango softens and becomes slightly caramelized. Taste and adjust seasoning with salt and pepper as needed.

3.**Assemble the Dish:** Return the chicken breasts to the skillet, spoon some of the mango jalapeno salsa over the top, and let it warm through for 2 minutes. (Cook time may differ depending on your rice brand; check instructions)

4.**Garnish and Serve:** Garnish with fresh cilantro if desired. Serve the chicken breasts with the mango jalapeño salsa on top of rice, quinoa, or a side of sautéed vegetables.

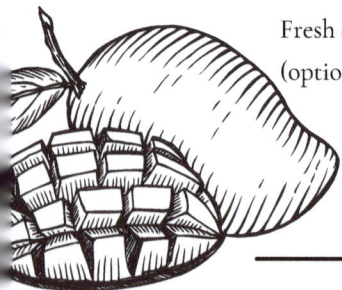

# Coconut Rice

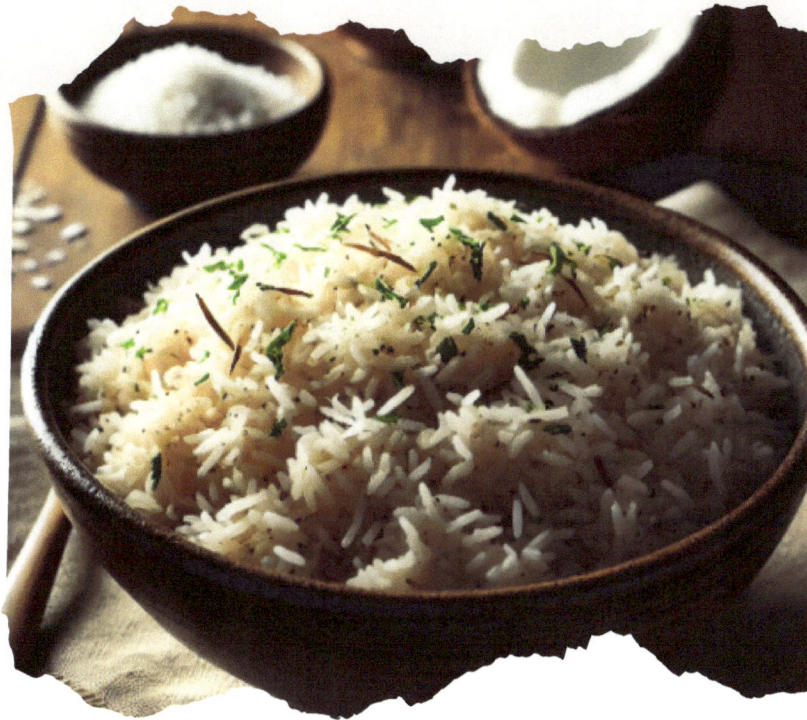

*This image may not be an accurate representation of the recipe.

## Ingredients

1 cup brown jasmine rice (or your preferred rice)

1 cup coconut milk
(full-fat for creamier rice)

1 cup water

1 tablespoon monk fruit sugar
(optional)

1/2 teaspoon salt

1 tablespoon olive oil or butter

## Method

1.**Rinse the Rice:** Rinse the rice under cold water until the water runs clear. This helps remove excess starch and prevents the rice from being too sticky.

2.**Cook the Rice:** In a medium saucepan, combine the rinsed rice, coconut milk, water, sugar (if using), and salt. Bring the mixture to a boil over medium-high heat.

3.**Simmer:** Once it boils, reduce the heat to low and cover the saucepan with a tight-fitting lid. Let it simmer for about 18-20 minutes or until the rice is tender and the liquid has been absorbed. Do not open the lid during cooking to keep the steam in.

4.**Fluff and Serve:** After the rice is cooked, remove it from the heat and let it sit, covered, for about 5 minutes. Fluff the rice with a fork and stir in a tablespoon of butter or olive oil if desired for extra flavor.

Goes well with the Jalapeno Mango Chicken Breast!

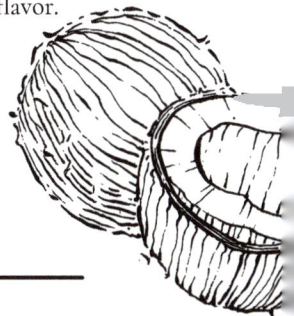

# Sautéed Squash

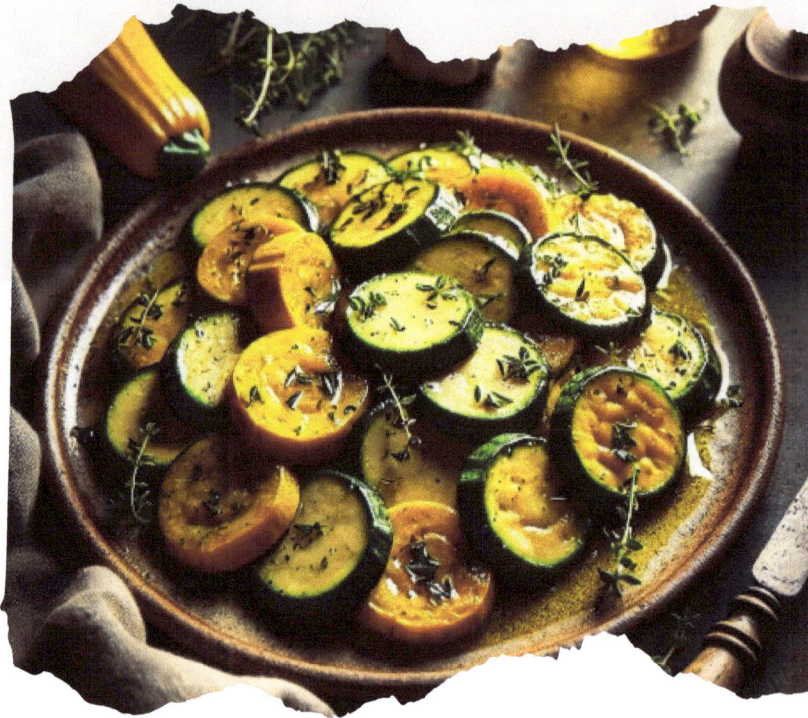

*This image may not be an accurate representation of the recipe.*

## Ingredients

2 medium zucchinis, sliced

2 medium yellow squash, sliced

2 tbsp olive oil

2 minced cloves garlic

Salt and pepper, to taste

1 tsp dried Italian seasoning

1/4 cup of chopped parsley

1 tablespoon of lemon juice

## Method

1.**Prepare the Vegetables:** Wash and slice the zucchini and yellow squash into 1/4-inch thick rounds or half-moons, depending on your preference.

2.**Heat the Pan:** Heat olive oil in a large skillet over medium heat. Add Garlic: Add the minced garlic to the pan and sauté in oil for 30 seconds, stirring, making sure it doesn't burn.

3.**Cook the Zucchini and Squash:** Add the sliced zucchini and yellow squash to the pan. Stir to coat the vegetables in the oil and garlic. Season and increase heat to medium-high Sauté for 5-7 minutes, stirring occasionally, until the squash and zucchini are tender but still slightly crisp.

4.**Add Lemon Juice:** Squeeze a little lemon juice over the vegetables before serving.

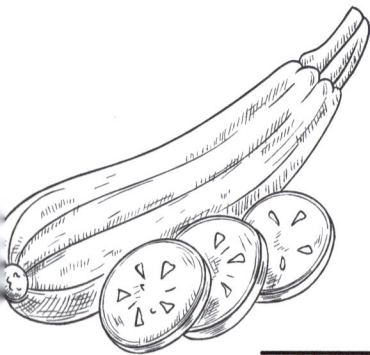

# Brown Rice Lo Mein

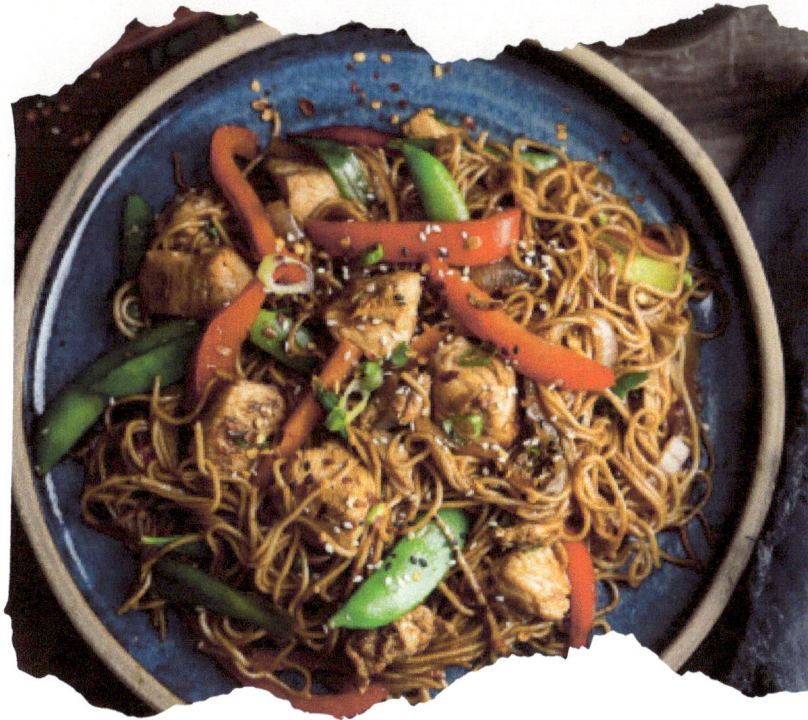

*This image may not be an accurate representation of the recipe.*

## Ingredients

8 oz brown rice pasta (spaghetti or linguine)

1 tbsp sesame oil

2 tbsp coconut aminos

1 tbsp rice vinegar

1 tbsp honey

1 minced garlic clove

1-inch piece of ginger, grated

1/2 onion julienne cut

cup mixed vegetables (carrots, bell peppers, mushrooms, snap peas, etc.)

2 green onions, chopped

Sesame seeds (optional for garnish)

## Method

1. **Cook the pasta:** Boil water in a large pot and cook the brown rice pasta according to the package instructions (usually around 7-10 minutes). Drain and set aside, reserving a little pasta water.

2. **Prepare the sauce:** In a small bowl, mix together the coconut aminos, rice vinegar and honey. Set aside.

3. **Sauté the vegetables:** Heat the sesame oil in a large skillet or wok over medium-high heat. Add julienne onion and 1/2 of green onion (reserve rest for garnish) and saute until soft. Add the garlic and ginger, sautéing for 1-2 minutes until fragrant. Add the mixed vegetables and stir-fry for 3-4 minutes until tender-crisp.

4. **Combine the pasta and sauce:** Add the cooked brown rice pasta to the skillet with the vegetables. Pour the sauce over the pasta and toss everything together.

5. **Finish and serve:** Stir in the green onions and cook for an additional 1-2 minutes. Garnish with green onions and a sprinkle of sesame seeds if desired.

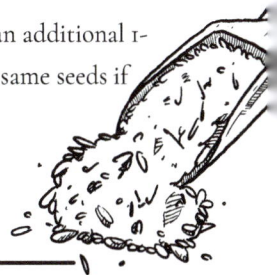

# Sweet Potato Medallions

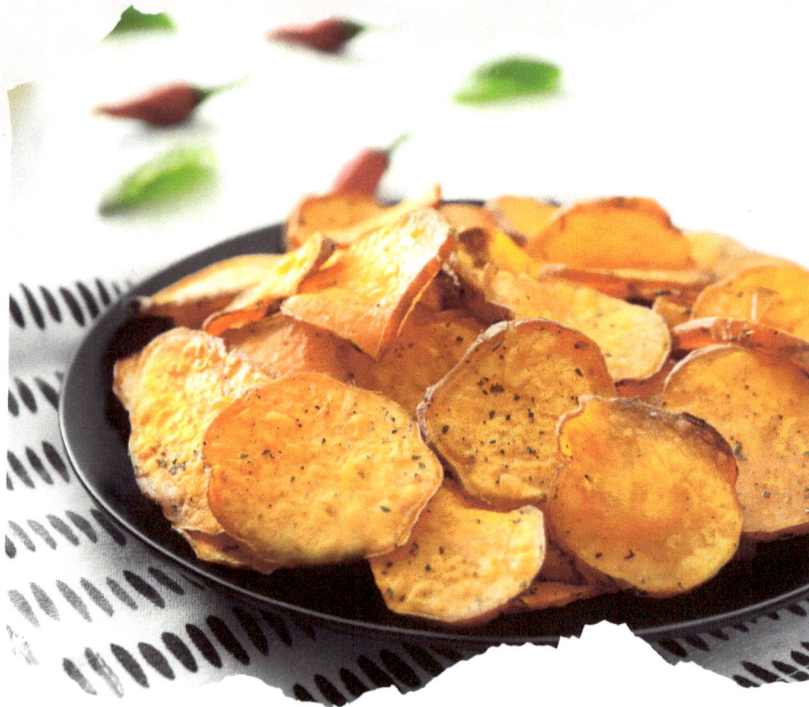

*This image may not be an accurate representation of the recipe.

## Ingredients

2 large sweet potatoes
2 tbsp olive oil
1 tsp garlic powder
1/2 tsp smoked paprika (optional)
Salt and pepper, to taste
Fresh herbs (like rosemary or thyme), optional

## Method

1.**Preheat the Oven:** Preheat your oven to 400°F. Line a baking sheet with parchment paper for easy cleanup.

2.**Prepare the Sweet Potatoes:** Peel the sweet potatoes and slice them into 1/2-inch thick rounds (medallions).

3.**Season the Medallions:** In a bowl, toss the sweet potato medallions with olive oil, garlic powder, smoked paprika (if using), salt, and pepper. Make sure each medallion is evenly coated.

4.**Arrange on the Baking Sheet:** Place the seasoned sweet potato medallions in a single layer on the prepared baking sheet.

5.**Roast the Medallions:** Roast the sweet potato medallions in the preheated oven for 20-25 minutes, flipping them halfway through to ensure they cook evenly. They should be tender on the inside and lightly browned on the outside.

6.**Top with Herbs:** Once they're done, sprinkle with fresh herbs like rosemary or thyme

**Great with the meatloaf!**

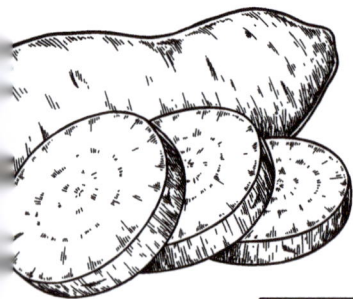

# Korean Beef

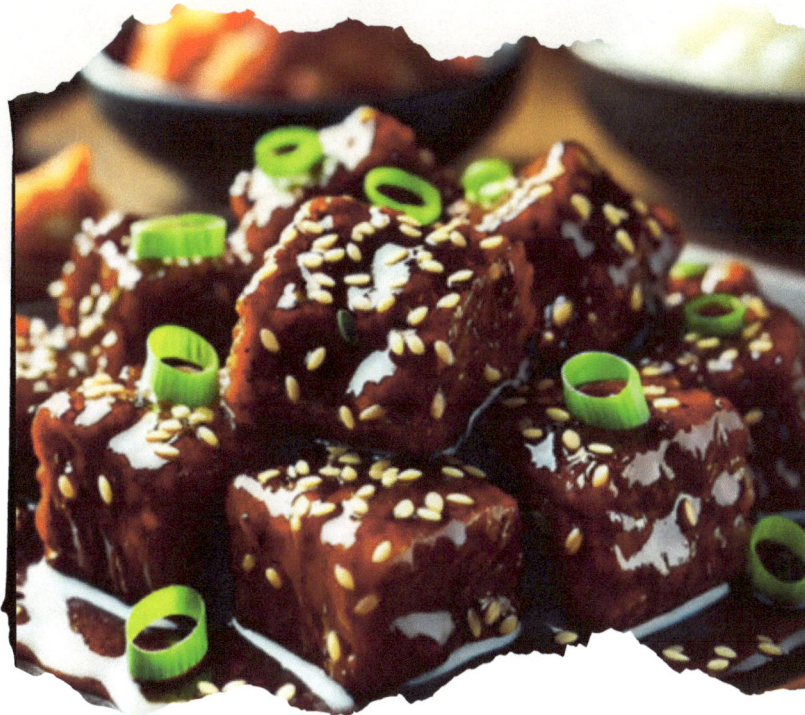

*This image may not be an accurate representation of the recipe.

## Ingredients

2 pounds beef sirloin cut into one-inch cubes

**For the Marinade:**

1 cup of coconut aminos in addition to 1/3 cup of coconut aminos

2 tbsp honey

2 tbsp sesame oil

1 tbsp minced garlic

1 tbsp grated ginger

1 tbsp rice vinegar or apple cider vinegar

1 tbsp gochujang (Korean red chili paste)

1 tbsp sesame seeds

2 green onions, chopped (plus more for garnish)

2 tsp cassava flour (optional, for thickening the sauce. Mix 3 tsp in 2 tbsp water to make a slurry, whisk in sauce on low heat)

Salt and pepper to taste

## Method

1.**Prepare the Beef:** Cut your beef into bite-sized cubes, making sure they are uniform in size for even cooking.

2.**Make the Marinade:** In a bowl, whisk together the coconut aminos or honey, sesame oil, minced garlic, grated ginger, rice vinegar, gochujang (if using), sesame seeds, and green onions.

Place the beef cubes in a resealable bag or shallow dish and pour the marinade over the meat. Seal the bag or cover the dish, and marinate in the fridge for at least 30 minutes, or ideally 2-4 hours for more flavor.

3.**Cook the Beef:** Heat a large skillet or wok over medium-high heat. If desired, add a little oil to the pan.

Add the marinated beef cubes to the pan, reserving some of the marinade for later. Sauté for 5-7 minutes, stirring occasionally, until the beef cubes are browned on all sides.

4.**Make the Sauce:** Add the reserved marinade and the cup of coconut aminos. Bring to a simmer. If you prefer a thicker sauce, you can add cassava flour slurry, stir it in and mix. Cook for another minute or so until the sauce thickens. Add salt and pepper to taste.

5.**Garnish and Serve:** Remove from heat and garnish with additional chopped green onions and sesame seeds.

Serve with steamed brown Jasmine rice or brown pasta rice lo mein

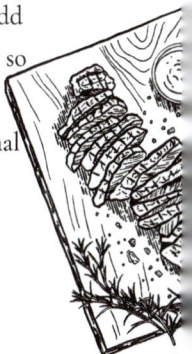

# Poblano Pineapple Chicken Enchiladas

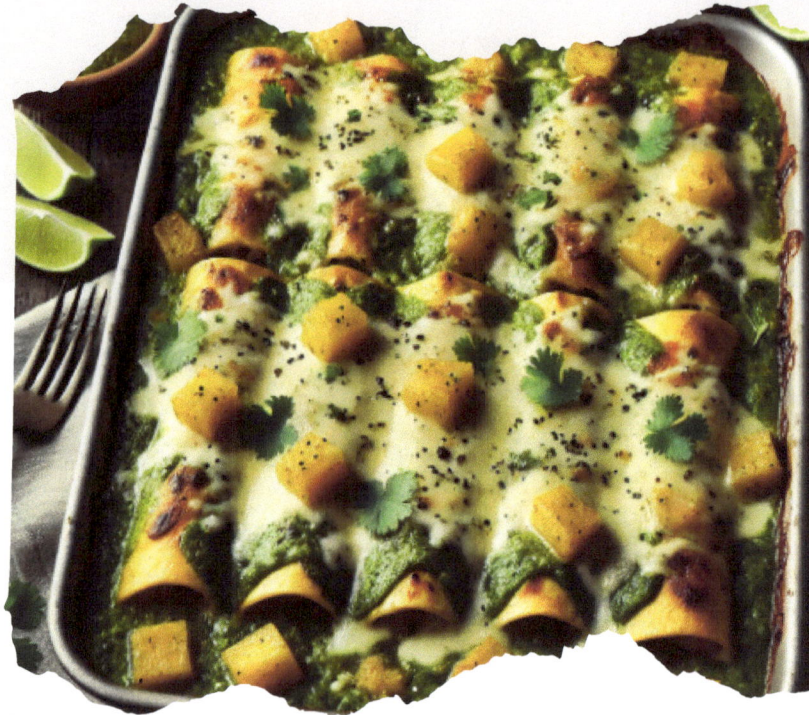

*This image may not be an accurate representation of the recipe.*

## Ingredients

**For the Chicken:**

2-3 pounds chicken breasts (or thighs)

1/2 onion, quartered

2 cloves garlic

1 bay leaf

Salt and pepper, to taste

**For the Green Sauce:**

4-5 medium tomatillos, husked and rinsed

2 poblano peppers, charred, peeled, and deseeded

1 small jalapeño (optional, for heat)

1/2 cup cilantro, chopped

A half of small, diced onion

1 tablespoon of cumin

2 cloves garlic

Juice of 1 lime

Salt and pepper, to taste

1/2 cup chicken broth or water

**For the Enchiladas:**

8 Siete cassava flour tortillas

2 cups shredded cooked chicken (from above)

1 1/2 cups shredded goat cheddar

Fresh cilantro, chopped (for garnish)

## Method

**1. Cook the Chicken:**

In a medium saucepan, add the chicken breasts, quartered onion, garlic cloves, bay leaf, salt, and pepper. Cover with water and bring to a boil. Once boiling, reduce the heat and simmer for 15-20 minutes until the chicken is cooked through.

Remove the chicken from the pot and shred it using two forks. Set aside. Saving the broth in the pot.

**2. Make the Green Sauce:**

Roast the tomatillos, poblano peppers, and jalapeño (if using) on a grill or in a dry skillet over medium-high heat, turning them occasionally until charred on all sides.

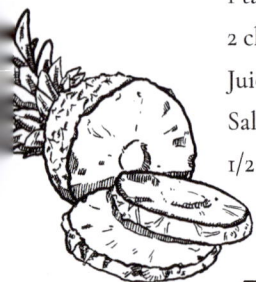

Once charred, place the poblano peppers in a bowl and cover with a towel to steam for 5 minutes, then peel and deseed them. In a blender, combine the roasted tomatillos, poblano peppers, jalapeño, cilantro, onion, garlic, lime juice, and chicken broth (from the pot) or water. Blend until smooth, and season with salt and pepper to taste.

### 3.Prepare the Tortillas:

In a skillet, lightly fry the siete tortillas in a small amount of oil just until they are soft and pliable (about 10-15 seconds per side). Alternatively, you can oil each side via spray and heat them in the microwave, wrapped in a towel for 20 seconds.

### 4.Assemble the Enchiladas:

Preheat your oven to 350°F

Spread a little bit of the green sauce on the bottom of a baking dish.

Take a tortilla, fill it with some shredded chicken, and roll it up. Place it seam-side down in the baking dish.

Repeat with the remaining tortillas and chicken.

### 5.Top the Enchiladas:

Once all the tortillas are in the dish, pour the remaining green sauce over the top of the enchiladas.

Shred the goat cheese evenly over the top.

### 6.Bake:

Bake the enchiladas for 20-25 minutes or until the cheese is melted and bubbly.

### 7.Serve:

Serve the enchiladas with a sprinkle of fresh cilantro on top.

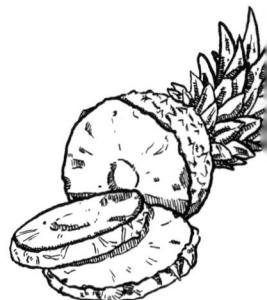

# Turkey Bacon BBQ Meatloaf

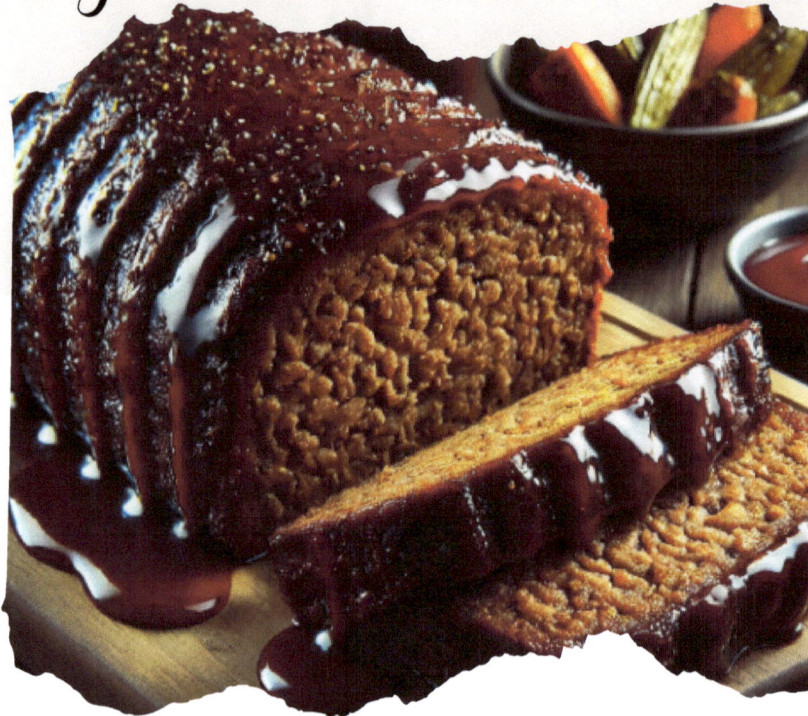

*This image may not be an accurate representation of the recipe.

## Ingredients

**For the Meatloaf:**

1 lb ground beef

1/2 lb turkey bacon, cooked and chopped

1 small red onion, finely chopped

1/2 cup green and red bell peppers chopped

1/4 cup chopped carrots

2 cloves garlic, minced

1 cup almond flour

1/4 cup water

1 large egg

1 tbsp Dijon mustard

1 tbsp Worcestershire sauce

1 tsp salt

1/2 tsp black pepper

1 tsp dried thyme or Italian seasoning

**For the BBQ Glaze:**

1 cup Primal Kitchen BBQ sauce (your favorite brand or homemade)

2 tbsp honey or swerve brown sugar (for a sweeter glaze)

## Method

1.**Preheat Oven:** Preheat your oven to 325°F

2.**Prepare the Meatloaf Mixture:** In a large bowl, combine the ground beef, chopped onion, chopped bell peppers, carrots, minced garlic, almond flour, water, egg, Worcestershire sauce, Dijon mustard, salt, pepper, and Italian seasoning. Mix until well combined.

3.**Form the Meatloaf:** Transfer the meat mixture into a greased loaf pan (or form a loaf shape on a lined baking sheet if you prefer).

4.**Prepare the BBQ Glaze:** In a small bowl, whisk together the BBQ sauce, honey or swerve brown sugar (if using) and turkey bacon. Taste and adjust as needed.

5.**Bake the Meatloaf:** Bake the meatloaf in the preheated oven for about 45-50 minutes, or until the internal temperature reaches 165°F

6.**Glaze and Rest:** Glaze the top of the meatloaf and let rest before slicing.

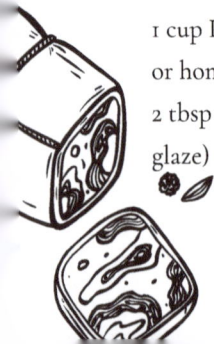

# Raspberry Loaf

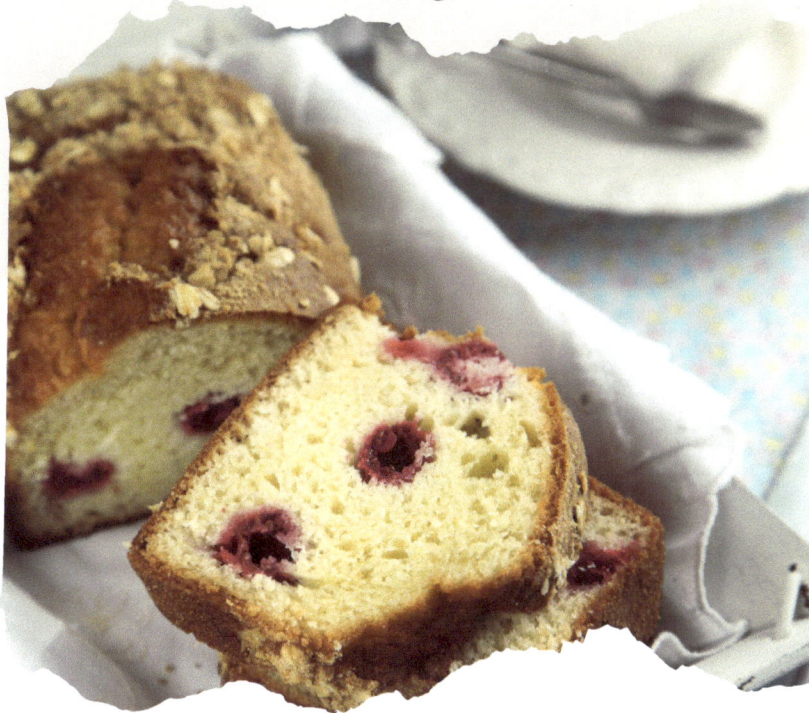

*This image may not be an accurate representation of the recipe.*

## Ingredients

4 eggs

1 small Lemon juiced

Lemon zest of 1 small lemon

1 tsp Vanilla

1/4 cup Monk fruit sugar

1/3 cup of melted coconut oil

1/2 tsp Baking soda

1/4 tsp salt

2 cups Almond flour

1/4 cup Coconut flour

1-pint Raspberries

## Method

1. **Preheat Oven:** Preheat oven to 325 degrees and oil loaf pan, then dust with almond flour.
2. **Mix Wet Ingredients:** Lightly beat eggs, then add lemon juice, lemon zest, sugar, vanilla and coconut oil.
3. **Mix Dry Ingredients:** In another bowl, mix coconut flour and almond flour together with baking soda.
4. **Add Dry Ingredients to Wet:** Add dry ingredients to the wet ingredients and mix until incorporated.
5. **Fold In Raspberries:** Add the raspberries and fold in gently. Pour into prepped loaf pan. Mix will be dry, but the moisture from raspberries with moisten it
6. **Bake:** Bake 35-40 min until a toothpick comes out clean
7. **Rest:** Rest the loaf on a cooling rack for 30 minutes before slicing

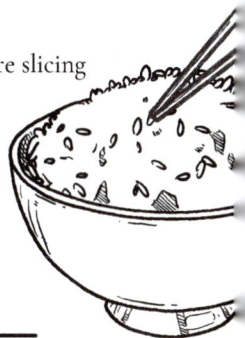

# Chocolate Cassava Pudding

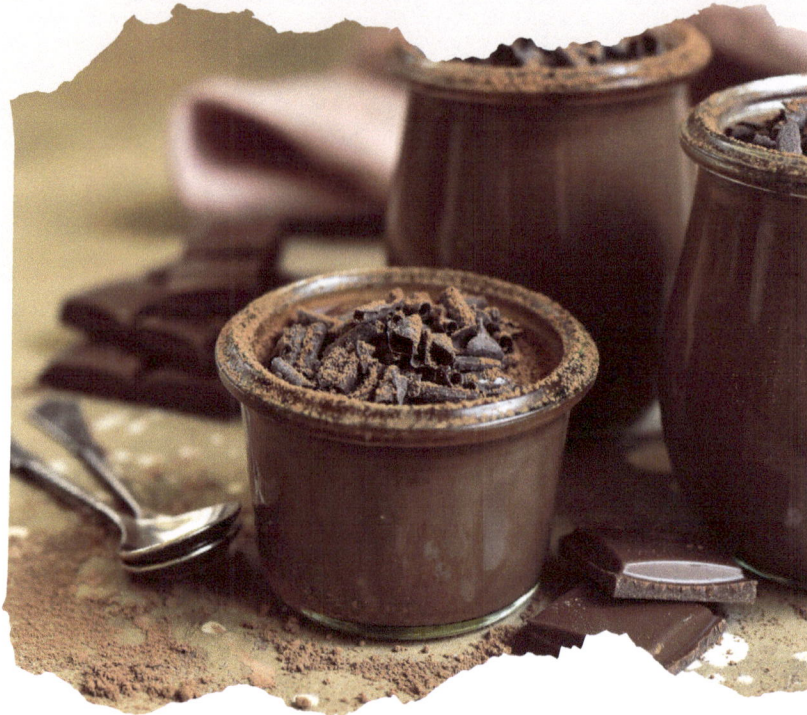

*This image may not be an accurate representation of the recipe.

## Ingredients

1/4 cup cassava flour

1/4 cup Monkfruit sugar

1/8 cup of agave nectar

1/4 cup unsweet cocoa powder

2 eggs

2 cups almond milk

1 tbsp butter

1 teaspoon vanilla

## Method

1.**Mix Dry Ingredients:** Add cassava flour, a Monk fruit sugar and cocoa powder, whisk to combine.

2.**Add Wet Ingredients:** Add eggs and mix until paste forms. Whisk in the milk until smooth.

3.**Cook:** Add mixture to a saucepan on medium heat. Continue to whisk until the mixture starts to thicken (do not leave because the egg will coagulate). Stir until the mix is thick enough to coat the back of a wooden spoon

4.**Add Butter and Vanilla:** Remove from heat and add the butter and vanilla. Mix in until melted.

5.**Portion:** Pour into a separate serving container or in a shallow dish and cover with plastic to prevent a film from forming on the top.

6.**Chill:** chill for at least an hour to set.

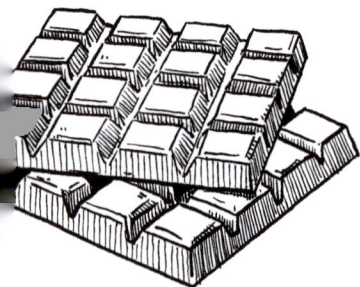